The Asthma Diet

by

Lynne D M Noble

All rights reserved. No part of this publication may be reproduced, stored in a retrieval system or transmitted in any form or by any means, without prior permission in writing of the author Lynne D M Noble, or as expressly agreed by law, or under terms agreed with the appropriate reprographics right organisation.

You must not circulate this book in any other binding or cover and you must impose the same condition on any acquirer.

Independently published 2019

Contents

Chapter	Page
About the author	iii
Preface	vi
Personal story	1
Asthma – an overview	6
Inflammation in asthma	9
The role of 5-lipoxygenase In the treatment of asthma	26
Natural suppressors of arachidonic acid and the D5D pathway	40
Inflammation, free radicals and antioxidants	55
Sugar and inflammation	66
Salicylates in food can contribute to asthma symptoms in some people	71
The asthma imposter	74
Theophylline	79
strategic response to the state of acidosis in order to reduce pain and inflammation	83
The dangers of MCA in the diet	94
The role of zinc deficiency	112
Medications which diminish vit C	121

DEDICATION

With many thanks to all the staff at the

Brinton Arms

Bewdley Road

Stourport-on-Severn

Where great service and good food has always been enjoyed

Keep Smiling ☺

About the Author

Lynne Noble was born in 1953 in Huddersfield, West Yorkshire. From a very early age, Lynne showed an interest in nutrition and genetics avidly reading any books that she could get her hands on at the time.

Initially, Lynne studied orthopaedics but events led her to work with the elderly mentally infirm. Here, her interest in neurodegenerative disorders and pain syndromes developed.

Lynne undertook rigorous programmes of study, completing her Cert Ed., (FE) BSc (Hons) and Adv. Dip Education simultaneously before moving onto her M.Ed.

From there she took further programmes of study in Human Nutrition, Pharmacology, Neuroscience, Genetics and Immunology. During this time, she was given many prestigious awards for her academic work. It was noted then that Lynne was not afraid of tackling difficult subjects.

She began her law degree but ill health prevented her from pursuing this. Nevertheless, she is active in upholding the rights of those with disabilities who are discriminated against.

She is a fan of the elderly and spent many years actively improving the lives of those in care homes.

In this time, she moved from being a foster parent to adoptive parent.

She has been instrumental in setting up projects in the community for disadvantaged groups.

Of particular importance was the BREAD initiative where groups of volunteers were trained to assist children who were failing in school. This achieved marked success.

She was nominated for the Yorkshire Television Outstanding Adult Learner Award 1992. She also was awarded the Yorkshire Open University

Graduates Educational Trust Award, among others.

Lynne is a member of the Guild of Health Writers and the British Union of Journalists.

Now retired, she lives in a picturesque village in West Yorkshire with her husband. She enjoys gardening, watching her husband bowling and researching.

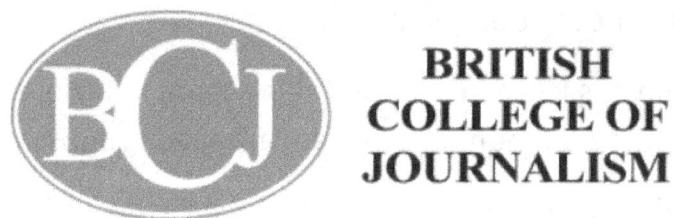

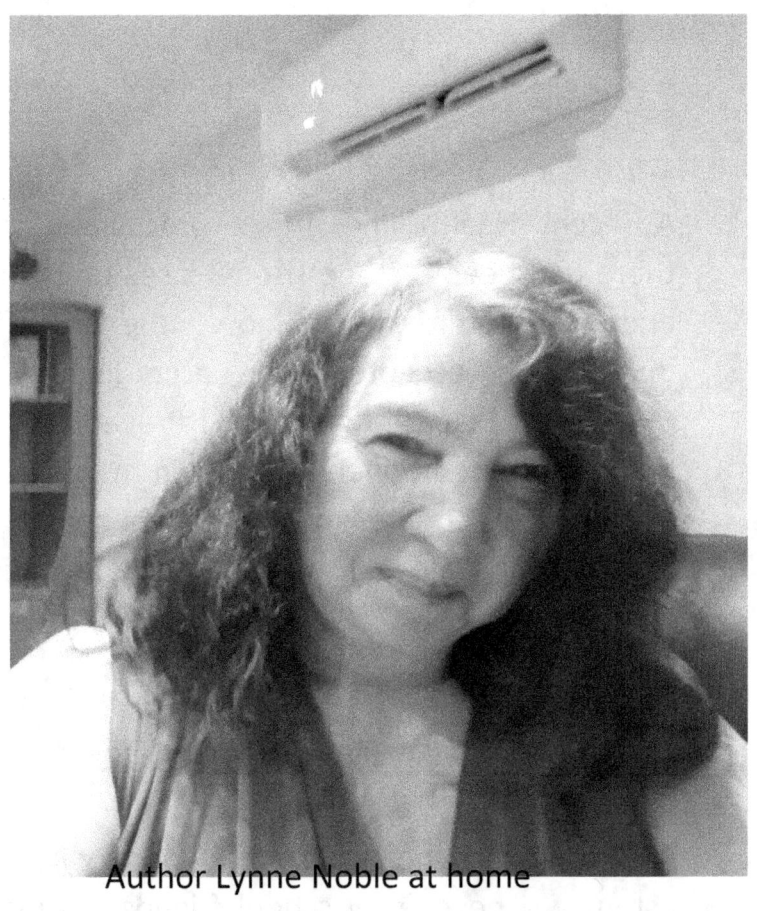

Author Lynne Noble at home

https://quintessentiallylynne.weebly.com/nutritional-medicine.html

author website:
https://www.amazon.co.uk/~/e/B07BPQZ5CD

Preface

A recent Health line article proclaimed that there had been a steep rise in cases of asthma and allergies in the U.S. over the past few decades. The accepted rate – according to the Centers for Disease Control and Prevention – is that about one in twelve people in the US have asthma. This equates to 25 million people or an increase of 28% of people who have this condition.

Nearer to my home, in the UK, ITV[1] news reported that asthma deaths have risen to their highest level in more than a decade.

As a child I did not know of anybody who had asthma. I never saw school friends having to use an inhaler. If people had asthma, it appeared to remain mild. Mine was mild, it did not stop me doing anything although I probably

---

[1] https://www.itv.com/news/2019-08-09/asthma-deaths-in-england-and-wales-rise-by-a-third-in-10-years/

did get more chest infections than my contemporaries.

It was only when I was nursing that I realised the severity of asthma. I was working on an orthopaedic ward at the time. A 17-year-old acquaintance had been admitted to another ward with status asthmaticus. A nurse on that ward came over to inform me of this and later to tell me that this young girl had died. It took a while to sink in.

What has changed in our society that has caused the increase in this debilitating condition? We know that pollution levels have risen considerably and this may be one obvious answer for *some* people. There are non-allergic types of asthma that are influenced by indoor and outdoor pollutants, cold air or exercise. Pollution increases free radicals and the antidote to this is to increase the amount of antioxidants in the diet. Indeed, this is good advice for any medical condition where inflammation is at the heart of it.

However, there are many more insidious causes of asthma that have not been explored. They are contained within our changing diets which promote substances that cause the symptoms of asthma. A number of sweeping changes to our diets have been made since the early 1900's but more so since the 1950's.

Not all cases of asthma-like symptoms are due to asthma. There is a condition with similar characteristics, that resembles bronchial asthma but needs to be recognised as a separate condition. This will be examined in some detail as it is not always recognised by medics.

As always, the remedies for medical conditions can generally be found within bespoke diets. As such, you will learn a little about the processes underpinning asthma and how just a few changes to diet can change the severity of the condition and lead to a more positive outcome.

Let us begin.

A way

It is a mystery to me
How you all breathe with such
consistency
I cannot hold a breath
I gasp in symphonies
I grasp at air running out my lungs

Lexie August 2017

Personal Story

I had mild asthma as a child - not that it was ever diagnosed then. We weren't encouraged to be ill in my house. It was considered a nuisance. This didn't stop me getting frequent bouts of tonsillitis and chest infections. It didn't stop me wheezing – especially when I laughed. It was only when I was older, and I was eventually diagnosed with asthma, that I learned that most of my maternal aunts and my maternal grandmother all had asthma.

One of my aunts recall my grandmother leaning out of the window gasping for breath. I wasn't that bad though. It didn't seem to stop my enjoyment of childhood. However, there was one bout that occurred when I was a young adult and had run, a short distance, for a bus. I couldn't draw breath into my lungs once I was on the bus. I thought that I would pass out. I didn't but I was exhausted once my breathing had recovered. Exhausted and a little concerned that it would happen again.

I hadn't been diagnosed with asthma at that point. It was not that I lacked exercise. I walked everywhere. To say that the roads in West Yorkshire are hilly was an understatement. I walked over three miles to work and then another three miles back. It usually did not present any problem.

I still continued to get chest infections though. I had small children to look after and couldn't afford to keep getting ill. I had just been promoted at work and was keen to make changes in the residential home I was working in.

It was a difficult time, many of my staff went down with flu.' I didn't at the beginning of the flu' epidemic. It was just as well since someone had to run the home. When I did eventually succumb to the virus, I rapidly became ill and sounded, according to my GP, like a steam engine.

I was despatched from the surgery with antibiotics, steroids, Alupent syrup and inhalers. I later found out that my notes said 'status asthmaticus'.

After a course of steroids and after the third course of antibiotics I was pronounced infection free. I was informed that as I had finished the course of steroids and antibiotics I must be well enough to return to work. The reality was that I was barely able to walk or think. During that time, I lay on the sofa, too weak to move. I only rose when the children came home from school. I would try and make them something to eat but often gave up as I could barely stand upright.

I was too breathless to walk up the stairs. I could only crawl up a couple at a time before needing to rest. Concerned friends picked me up and took me out for some sun. They poured Instant Whip down my throat – I was far too exhausted to eat. Even sipping a cup of tea was exhausting.

I gave up work. I wasn't fit to look after myself, never mind thirty-seven challenging residents.

If I had been given a peak flow meter, then the problem would have been clear. I wasn't given one though. In fact, I wasn't given a peak flow meter until 2009 – that is more than 30 years after that experience.

Now I recognise the symptoms of a low peak flow but I wish that I'd known years ago. I wish that I had known that a low peak flow would give me brain fog or make my limbs heavy or account for my need to go to bed early because I was so tired. I wish that I had known that it would be difficult to think or concentrate on simple things. I wish my GP had realised that just because the infection had gone it did not mean that my lungs were not inflamed and that breathing would be difficult until this sorted itself out.

I worked this all out eventually. I was in my mid-fifties before someone explored whether asthma might be responsible for my constant chest infections. Yes, I had a diurnal rhythm. It explained why I would wake up gasping for air in the middle of the night. That had been ongoing for years and had become the norm for me.

I was given two inhalers originally but then the two were merged into one. I'm not keen on anything steroid based. Steroids lower immunity and they thin your skin. I have heard all the arguments about inhaled steroids remaining in the lungs and not exerting a systemic effect. This did not explain why my stomach blew up like a balloon when I used the inhalers and why this phenomena went when I stopped using them.

At times of severe infection, I would be prescribed steroids. These left me mentally fragile. My blood sugars went up dramatically and I was placed in a diabetic state.

Steroids are renowned for their ability to cause dramatic weight gain and I was not denied this experience. The problems with steroids – apart from their ability to lower immunity and thin skin – is that they make tendons brittle so that they tear easily. For those with an underlying connective tissue disorder this is clearly of grave concern. I have hypermobile joints and thin veins. I did not want my connective tissue to become even more compromised or my veins to become any more fragile than they already were.

It became a quest to find a solution to the problem that I had. Luckily, my extensive background in research came in useful. I now still carry an inhaler around 'just in case' but I haven't had to use it for a number of years. My chest infections belong to the past. I still have a genetic propensity to asthma but environmental factors have effectively smothered its influence.

A genetic propensity to medical conditions like asthma does not mean that it HAS to manifest itself. Environmental factors will have the deciding factor in whether, or how it will be played out in life. So let's start in investigating the causes of asthma.

Asthma – an overview

Asthma is characterised by wheezing, breathlessness, fatigue, chest tightness and sleeplessness as well as increased risk of respiratory infections.

The 'twitchy' lungs, found in asthmatics, are overly sensitive and readily constrict in response to factors such as:

- Cold air
- Smoke
- Exercise
- Infection – even mild ones.
- allergens

Exercise can induce asthma

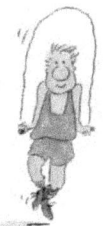

This can be useful to know if it helps us avoid likely triggers. However, it does not tell us about the underlying causes of asthma and what else we can do to prevent it affecting our lives. That is what this book is going to explore.

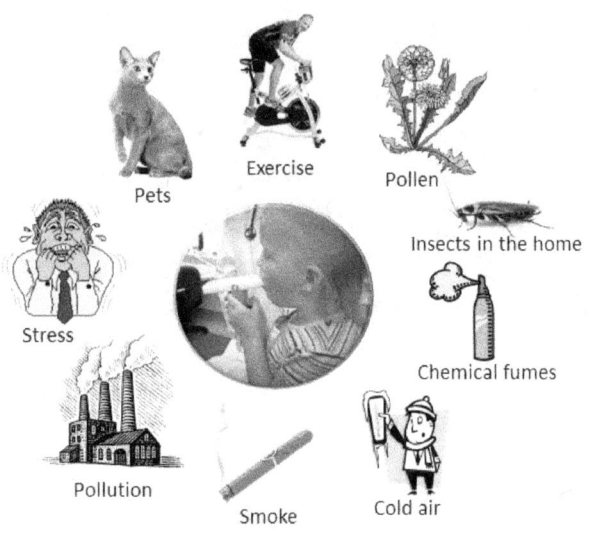

Asthma Triggers

Asthma occurs when the airways become inflamed. When they become inflamed they become narrower and it is harder to push air through the tubes. This causes the wheezing sound. Stickier mucous is produced and there is increased vascular permeability.

What happens when the tubes become inflamed? What exactly is causing that particular process?

Inflammation in asthma

In asthma a particular inflammatory substance has been found to be elevated. It is a leukotriene called leukotriene B4 (LTB4).

A leukotriene is a molecule that brings about inflammation.

When LTB4 levels are elevated then inflammation of the tissues occurs and this impairs the function of lung tissue.

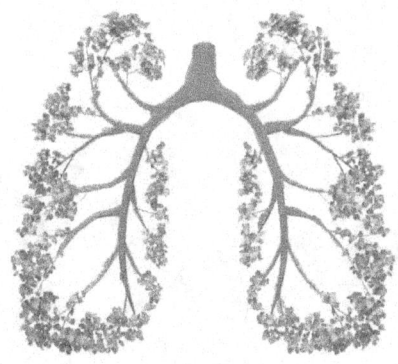

Elevated LBT4 levels cause inflammation in the lungs.

Some drugs are specifically made to target this disease process. That is, they inhibit the pathways that make LTB4. Some of these common inhalers are known as:

- Monteleukast
- Zafirlukast
- pranlukast

These drugs have many side effects such as:

- skin rash
- mood changes
- tremors
- headache
- stomach pain
- heartburn
- nausea

This is not a definitive list.

Since asthma is a chronic disease the continuing use of an inhaler - such as Monteleukast – with all its potential negative side effects, is likely.

The good news is that there are many nutrients which can also inhibit LTB4. However, we need to examine what leukotrienes actually are, in more detail.

Leukotrienes

The biochemical definition is:

Any of a group of biologically active compounds, originally isolated from leucocytes (white blood cells). They are metabolites of arachidonic acid, containing three conjugated bonds.

That's a bit of a mouthful so let's pull it apart and see what it really means.

A **leucocyte** is simply a white blood cell. They protect the body against infectious disease and foreign invaders.

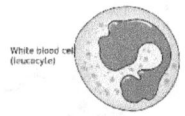

A **metabolite** is the very end product of some chemical processes that occur in a living organism, in order to maintain life.

Leukotrienes are the end product of **arachidonic acid.**

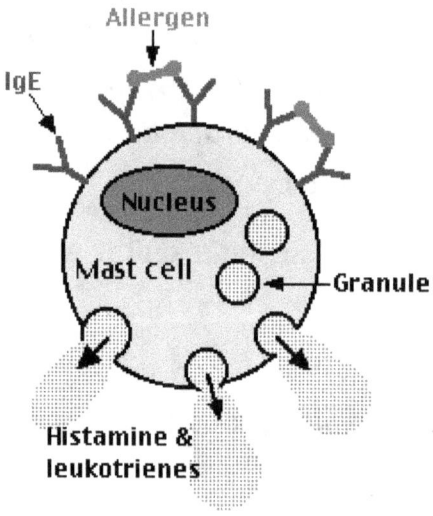

Arichidonic acid is a polyunsaturated omega-6 fatty acid. It is found in the membranes of the body's cells and is particularly abundant in the brain, muscles and liver. It is a key inflammatory intermediate and can act as a vasodilator. This means it can widen blood vessels.

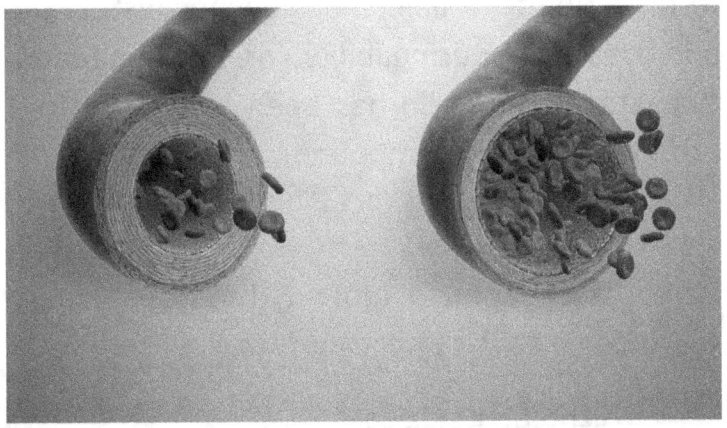

Second picture shows vasodilation. The vessel becomes thinner and leakier.

Arichidonic acid has many beneficial roles in the body. It will not cause inflammation unless tiny particles, called electrons, try and disrupt the stability of other electrons found in the fat that forms part of the cell membranes. Unfortunately, our current diets contain a lot of foods that do contain a lot of unpaired electrons. We will look at this shortly.

Arachidonic acid can be metabolised to both anti-inflammatory and pro-inflammatory eicanosoids. It is quite likely that if you suffer from joint pain, bronchoconstriction, microvascular permeability or lymphoedema that arachidonic acid has been converted to a pro-inflammatory compound.

Here are some more diseases where arachidonic acid is implicated.
- Alzheimer's disease
- Diabetes mellitus
- High blood pressure
- Cardiovascular disease
- Some cancers
- Mental health disorders
- Other respiratory disorders

In fact, many of the diseases that currently afflict society.

What is arachidonic acid exactly?

Arachidonic acid is a poly unsaturated omega 6 fatty acid. Most vegetable oils contain omega 6 fatty acids. Normally, arachidonic acid is required during or after physical activity. It helps to promote growth and cell repair when this is needed.

Although factors such as:

- Heavy metals
- Smoking
- Air pollution

are thought to be the main contributors to the development of asthma there is an association between the high intake of omega-6 fatty acids that are found in vegetable oils that are commonplace in kitchens. This is thought to be due to lipid peroxidation.

Lipid peroxidation occurs when free radicals (the unpaired electron) steal another electron from the lipids in cell membranes. Electrons simply do not like being unpaired and will wreak havoc knocking off electrons from other cells which they can pair up with. However, the consequences of this behaviour, is cell damage.

The body is clever. It requires repair but to do this inflammation must occur. The process of inflammation brings healing substances to the site of injury. Hopefully, the damage will be sorted out and resolution will occur.

However, our diets are now besieged with products containing hidden omega 6 fatty acids. We have replaced the saturated – and stable – fats that we used to eat and replaced them with vegetable oils that are easily oxidised and subsequently, cause damage to tissue This leaves us, more or less in a permanent inflammatory state.

The stable saturated fats are foods such as butter, lard and dripping. We used to eat them in abundance and did not suffer from inflammatory conditions to the extent that we do now.

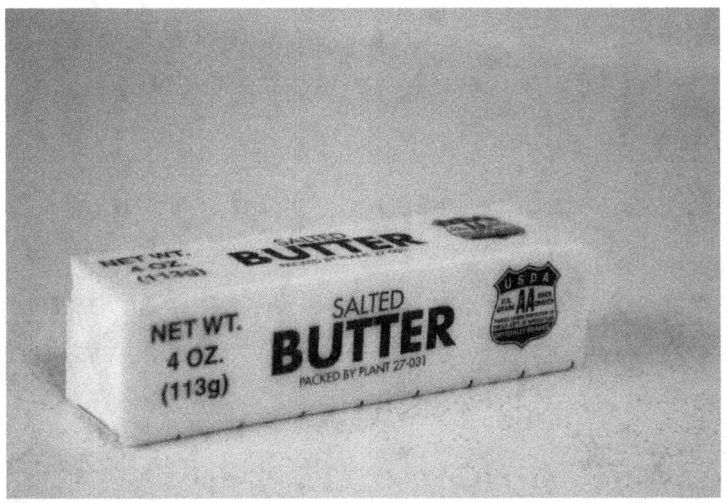

Before 1920 cardiovascular conditions, for example, were very low in the USA as they were in the UK. The Victorians, who ate a very high fat diet, suffered from so little heart disease, that it was not considered worth teaching about at medical school.

The saturated fats were a major source of vitamin D whereas vegetable oils do not contain any worth considering.

A new Cochrane review[2] has found evidence from randomised trials that supplementing with vitamin D – in addition to standard asthma medication – is likely to reduce severe asthma attacks.

Other studies[3] found that vitamin D supplements reduced the risk of asthma exacerbations by 26%. However, this protective effect was only seen in those who were vitamin D deficient in the first place.

A study[4] in Canada involving people aged 13-69 years found that those with vitamin D levels below 50 nmol/l (20ng/ml) were 50% more

---

[2] https://uk.cochrane.org/news/high-quality-evidence-suggests-vitamin-d-can-reduce-asthma-attacks

[3] https://www.nhs.uk/news/heart-and-lungs/vitamin-d-supplements-may-prevent-asthma-worsening-some/

[4] *Niruban, S.J., Alagiakrishnan, K., Beach, J., et al., Association between vitamin D and respiratory outcomes in Canadian adolescents and adults. J Asthma, 2015: p. 1-33.*

likely to have current asthma than those with levels between 20 and 30 ng/mol.

Approximately 80% of the world population are vitamin D deficient so levels of this vitamin need to be ascertained and remedied, if needed, in anyone who has asthma.

Why might vitamin D impact on the severity of asthma?

Vitamin D helps to synthesise an antimicrobial called cathelicidin which helps fight infection. In addition, Vitamin D helps regulate the immune system so that it works at its optimum level. Vitamin D prevents the body from going into 'inflammatory overdrive'. It is the key regulatory vitamin.

There are very few sources of vitamin D outside the saturated fats. They include:

- Oily fish
- Egg yolks
- Irradiated mushrooms

- Liver

Most of these foods are not usually liked by children. They are eaten far less than they used to be by all groups.

Another source of vitamin D is sunlight but only from the months of May to September in our climate.

In the 1950's children used to be given a daily dose of cod liver oil to prevent rickets. It may also help explain, in part, why asthma levels were much lower than they are now.

How ubiquitous are omega 6 fatty acids in our diet?

Omega 6 fatty acids are contained in just about any processed food that you can buy. My tin of 'healthy' baked beans contains rape seed oil. My favourite curry sauce does. The crackers that I eat also contain vegetable oil. About 90% of my emergency store cupboard items contain vegetable oil. Yes, it is ubiquitous. Here are some of the foods where they are hidden as well as some of the other most commonly consumed omega-6 rich foods.

- Mayonnaise
- Grapeseed oil
- Margarine
- Fast food
- Popcorn
- Restaurant food
- Salad dressing
- Rice bran oil
- Potato chips
- Granola
- Shortening
- Baked goods
- Peanut butter
- Bread
- Tortilla chips
- sauces

The ratio of omega 6 fatty acids to the omega 3 fatty acids (found in fish oil and walnuts) should be in the ratio of 1:6. In reality, it is the other way around. We are being force fed unsaturated fatty acids that oxidise easily, cause cell damage - and consequently inflammation - on a daily basis.

Percentage of Omega-6s and Omega-3s in Common Vegetable Oils

Oil	Omega-6s	Omega3s
Safflower	75%	0%
Sunflower	65%	0%
Corn	54%	0%
Cottonseed	50%	0%
Soybean	51%	7%
Peanut	32%	0%
Canola	20%	9%

[5]

---

[5] https://blog.biotrust.com/what-are-omega-6-fatty-acids/

Researchers[6] estimate that the average person's consumption of soybean oil increased more than 1000 fold from the early 1900's to the beginning of the 21st century.

By now we should have learned that omega 6 fatty acids are eaten in far greater amounts than omega 3 fatty acids. Therefore, our diet is pro inflammatory in nature.

Arachidonic acid - an omega 6 fatty acid - is implicated in the development of asthma.

Saturated fats are stable, do not contain omega 6 fatty acids and do not readily cause inflammation.

Saturated fats contain vitamin D and vitamin D has been found to reduce the severity of asthma attacks in those who are deficient in this vitamin.

---

[6] https://www.ncbi.nlm.nih.gov/pubmed/21367944

Therefore, useful changes in your diet are:

- Replace vegetable oils with the stable saturated fats
- Check vitamin D levels and supplement when necessary.

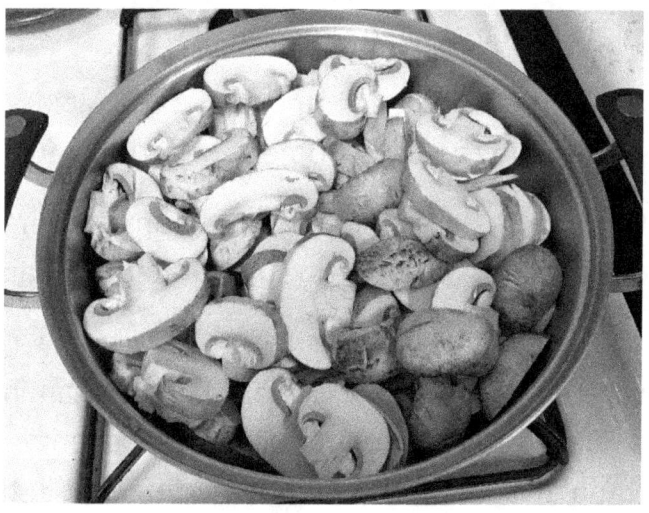

Mushrooms contain vitamin D

The role of 5-lipoxygenase (5-LO) inhibitors in the treatment of asthma

5-LO is an enzyme. It is required for the synthesis of leukotrienes responsible for asthma attacks.

Leukotrienes are molecules found in immune cells. Their main function is to promote inflammation. They do this by activating the production of inflammatory cells such as neutrophils and monocytes. Leukotrienes also activate molecules (cytokines) which are involved in inflammation.

There are two families of leukotrienes. The group we are interested in has the grand sounding name of cysteinyl-leukotrienes. These leukotrienes are concerned with eosinophil and mast cell induced bronchoconstriction.

In the more severe and chronic forms of asthma, the hyper-reactivity of the bronchial tubes is primarily caused by eosinophils. They are attracted to the bronchioles by the leukotrienes.

We shall look at eosinophils in more detail later.

5-LO is part of the first two steps necessary for the transformation of arachidonic acid to leukotrienes.

There is a clinically approved inhibitor of 5-LO called Zileuton. However, it has some unacceptable side effects.

Fortunately, there are some naturally occurring 5-LO inhibitors. These include:

- Bee propolis
- Hypericum perforatum
- Curcumin
- Gamma and Delta tocopherol (forms of vitamin E)
- Monoenoic acids
- Pumpkin seed

Honey bee propolis is:

- Anti-inflammatory in action
- Antiviral
- Anticancer
- Antibacterial

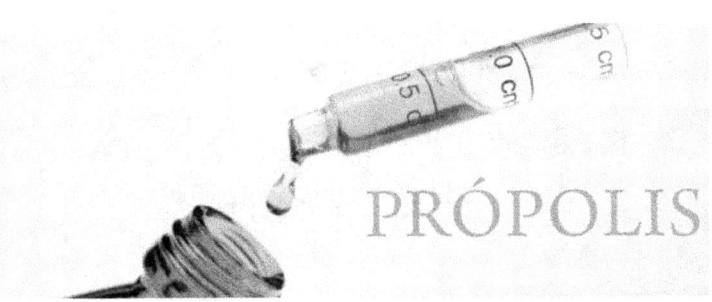

Diagram showing the process of conversion by the enzyme 5-lipoxygenase to inflammatory mediators

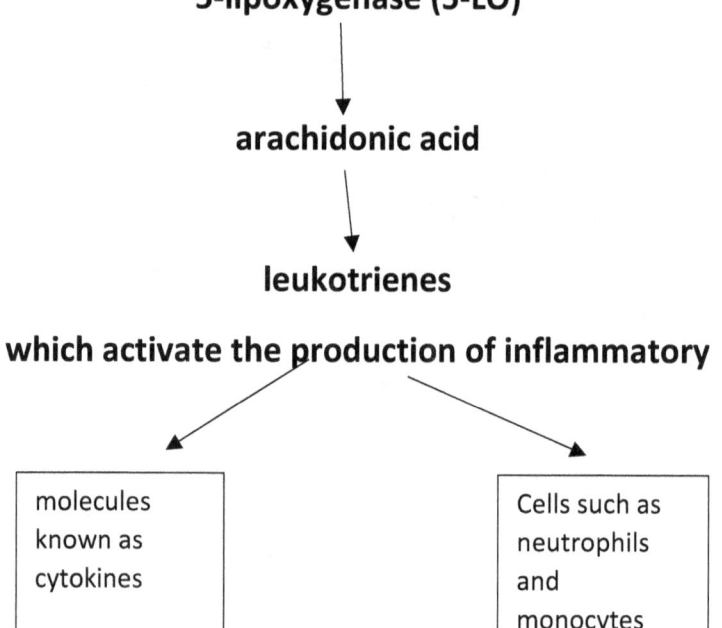

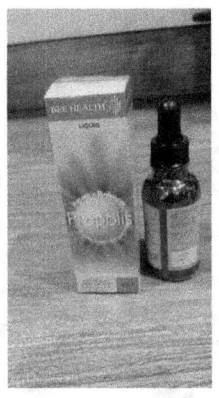

Monoenoic Fatty Acids

A number of long chain monoenoic fatty acids were found to have an effect on 5-LO activity. However, oleic acid found in olive oil has by far the greatest inhibitory effect on 5-LO.

Oleic acid is a monounsaturated fatty acid that is found in useful amounts in olive oil and macadamia nuts.

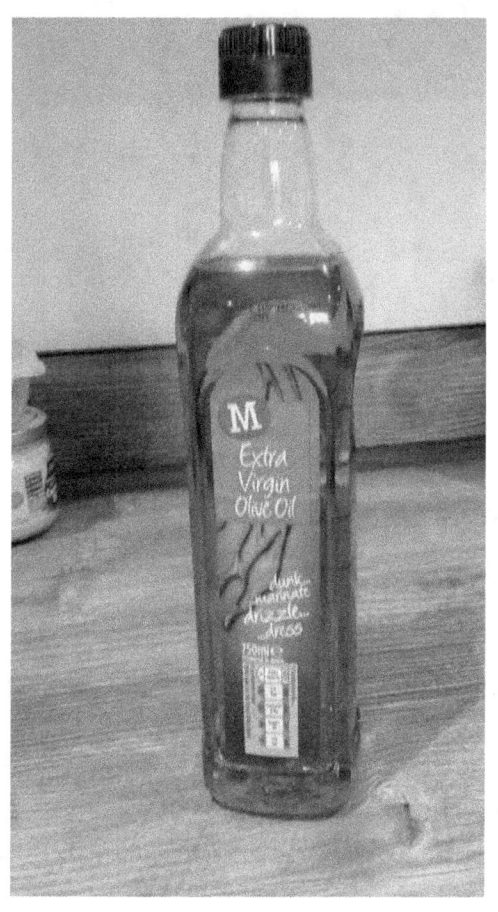

Dipping bread into olive oil, adding it to soups and making salad dressings with it are all useful habits to get into. Try and include it into your diet every day.

Lycopene and saw palmetto

Studies[7] have also shown that lycopene and saw palmetto extract also help to suppress 5-LO.

Lycopene is the antioxidant that gives tomatoes their red colour. The Mediterranean diet contains fresh fruit and vegetables with plenty of olive oil. It is a diet which would benefit those who have asthma.

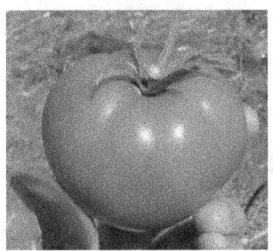

Caffeic acid is another 5-LO inhibitor which is found in a wide range of foods. Its main source is coffee but its name 'caffeic' has absolutely nothing to do with caffeine.

---

[7] Agarwal S, Rao AV. Tomato lycopene and its role in human health and chronic diseases. CMAJ. 2000 Sep 19;163(6):739-44.

Good sources of caffeic acid are:

- Wine[8]
- Turmeric
- Coffee
- Herbs such as basil, oregano, sage, thyme
- Apples
- Cabbage
- Strawberries
- Mushrooms
- Cauliflower
- Kale
- Pears
- Olive oil

---

[8] Some people may have allergies to other substances in red wine such as the sulphites that they contain.

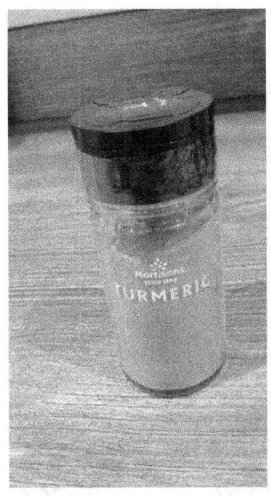

The active ingredient in turmeric, curcumin, is a 5-LO inhibitor.

Hypericum perforatum

A study[9] has found that naturally occurring analogues of hyperforin, that are isolated from H, perforatum, showed that oxidised hyperforin has efficacy against 5-LO.

The study was conducted on intact human polymorphnuclear leukocytes – a type of white blood cells.

---

[9] https://www.ncbi.nlm.nih.gov/pubmed/16787324

Hypericum perforatum can be obtained from supermarkets and health food stores.

Vitamin E

Studies[10] have shown that the end products of vitamin E limit inflammation by targeting 5-LO.

Vitamin E is actually a mixture of eight naturally derived substances. They are fat soluble antioxidants that help to prevent the damage that occurs in asthma. However, they also have anti-inflammatory effects which are not attributed to their antioxidant properties.

A vitamin E deficiency can result in severe degenerative disease, atherosclerosis and a poor immune response. It was found that when alpha tocopherol was supplemented above the recommended daily allowance which is 400 IU's then there was a marked anti-inflammatory, anti-atherosclerotic and anti- tumour efficacy.

This study was carried out on animals.

---

[10] https://www.nature.com/articles/s41467-018-06158-5

There are three types of vitamin E whose metabolites show good efficacy against 5-LO. These are:

- Gamma tocopherol
- Delta tocopherol
- Gamma tocotrienol

Some of the metabolites of vitamin E are shown in the table overleaf.

Pumpkin seeds also contain vitamin E and this may account for their inhibitory action on lipoxygenase.

Table[11] showing some of the inhibitory activity of vitamin E derivatives against 5-LO in cell-free and cell based test systems.

---

[11] https://www.nature.com/articles/s41467-018-06158-5/tables/1

	T				TE		
	α(a)	β(b)	γ(c)	δ(d)	α(e)	β(f)	γ(g)
Human recombinant 5-LO							
Vitamin E (1)	>1	0.75±0.15	0.91±0.15	0.31±0.10	0.33±0.08	0.19±0.03	0.20±0.06
13'-CH2-OH (2)	0.35±0.04			0.12±0.04	0.11±0.01	0.09±0.03	
12a-CH2-OH (3)							0.12±0.03
13'-COOH (4)	0.27±0.01			>1	0.46±0.06	0.15±0.04	0.30±0.10
Activated PMNL							
Vitamin E (1)	808±159	57±2	502±199	85±5	277±90	95±5	132±33
13'-CH2-OH (2)	0.19±0.05			0.54±0.02	0.27±0.10	0.38±0.09	
12'a-CH2-OH (3)							0.14±0.02
13'-COOH (4)	0.08±0.00			2.01±0.59	1.70±0.52	0.31±0.11	0.49±0.03

IC_{50} values (μM) are given as mean ± s.e.m. $n = 3$ independent experiments.

Wheat germ contains good amount so vitamin E

Sources of vitamin E

The best sources of vitamin E are:

- Seeds – sesame, sunflower. For example
- Nuts – almonds, hazelnuts, peanuts
- Vegetable oils – wheat germ, corn, soybean, safflower, for example. However, these oils are oxidised easily and, in doing so will produce inflammation. Keep oils cool and in the dark and use only once if you must use an omega 6 oil.
- Green leafy vegetables such as kale, spinach, chard and broccoli.

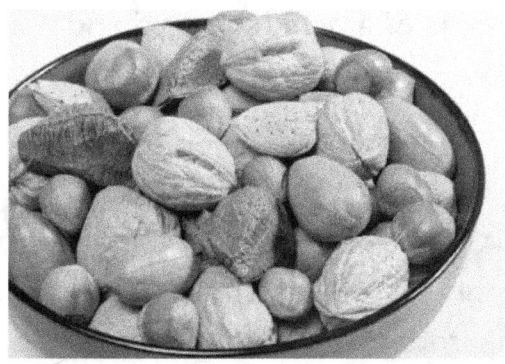

Nuts are an excellent source of vitamin E

Natural suppressors of arachidonic acid and the D5D pathway

Adenosine is a natural suppressor of arachidonic acid release and leukotriene biosynthesis. A potent natural source of adenosine is brewer's yeast. However, it competes with protein for absorption so it is better taken before food. As it also makes you feel sleepy – it is an inhibitory neurotransmitter – the perfect time to take it is before bedtime.

Copper is required for the synthesis of adenosine triphosphate which is required in every cell in the body.

Foods which contain copper include:

- Liver
- Oysters
- Nuts and seeds
- Lobster
- Dark leafy greens
- Dark chocolate

The recommended dietary allowance is 900mcg daily. However, a word of caution is required here – a deficiency or excess of copper can have negative side effects so supplementation is not recommended unless under medical supervision.

Further, if copper is not bound to a protein – which occurs in food as a matter of course – then it has toxic properties.

For example, the copper found in supplements is generally a salt of copper – that is an unbound form. I cannot recommend supplements of copper unless you know for certain that they are in a non-labile form.

Copper from copper pipes used to convey drinking to households is also toxic and should be avoided. The best sources of copper are from food in a well-balanced diet.

Signs of a copper deficiency include:

- abnormal skin and hair pigmentation
- iron deficient anaemia
- poorly functioning immune system resulting in bacterial infections
- poor memory and lack of creative thinking.

Eicosapentaenoic Acid

There is an omega 3 fatty acid called EPA (Eicosapentaenoic Acid) that inhibits the enzyme[12] [13] that produces arachidonic acid. The

---

[12] This enzyme is delta-5-desaturase (D5D)

[13] Sears B. The Zone. Regan Books. New York, NY (1995)

more EPA that you have in your diet the less arachidonic acid you will synthesise.

In effect EPA reduces the amount of arachidonic acid and subsequently the pro-inflammatory prostaglandins, thromboxanes, eicosanoids and leukotrienes.

In a nutshell:

EPA reduces the synthesis of arachidonic acid by inhibiting the enzyme D5D.

Reduced arachidonic acid = fewer inflammatory chemicals such as

- prostaglandins
- thromboxanes
- eicosanoids
- leukotrienes

So to reduce leukotrienes we can now target two pathways:

1) The pathway that synthesises arachidonic acid by making sure that we have plenty of EPA in the diet and
2) The pathway that makes LTB4 leukotrienes from arachidonic acid by including 5-LO inhibitors in the diet.

DHA, another omega three fatty acid and closely associated with EPA does not have this effect. It is not an inhibitor of the D5D enzyme. It has a greater spatial size and cannot compete with arachidonic acid for the enzyme phospholipase A2 that helps release arachidonic acid from the cell membrane phospholipids where it is stored. Only EPA can do this.

Interestingly, steroid therapy generally inhibits this D5D enzyme to reduce inflammation. However, EPA can do this too but without the numerous side effects of steroids.

The main source of EPA is oily fish such as salmon, pilchards, mackerel and sardines. Oily fish needs to be eaten daily – or cod liver oil capsules taken - when asthma is present. Failing this, supplementation is necessary as a preventative step in inhibiting the D5D enzyme that is necessary for the synthesis of arachidonic acid.

EPA, found in oily fish, is necessary in the battle against the synthesis of arachidonic acid and asthma.

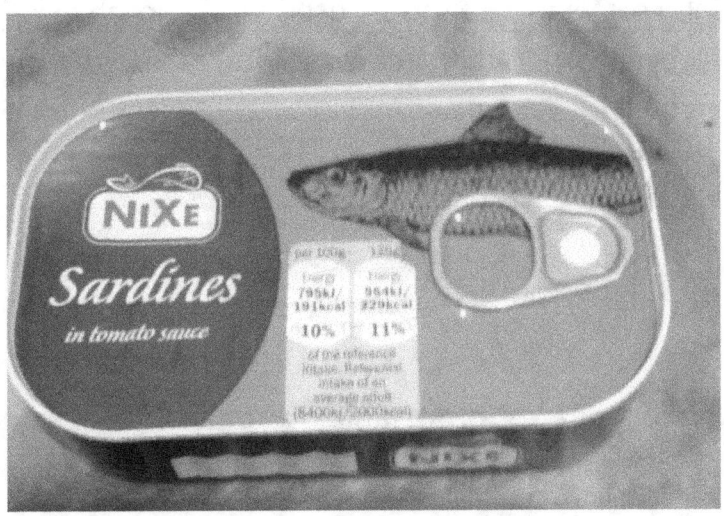

Cod liver oil is a great source of EPA, too.

Natural bronchodilators

Theophylline is often prescribed for those with asthma. It helps to alleviate breathlessness by relaxing muscles that cause constriction in the airways. Once they have opened up air is able to move through the tubes freely.

Coffee has been found to have a similar action of a duration of up to four hours. However, its onset of action is not as rapid as that found in inhalers so has more use as a prophylaxis (preventer) rather than as a rapid rescue remedy.

Coffee dilates bronchioles and enable easier breathing.

Magnesium

Magnesium has so many functions that its benefits should be more widely sung. It has an anti-inflammatory action and is beneficial for the inflammation found in the lungs of asthmatics. Magnesium is also an excellent anti-spasmodic alleviating the 'twitchiness' found in the bronchioles that constricts tubes making the passage of air difficult. This contributes to the wheezing characteristic of asthma.

Magnesium sulphate is used intravenously in severe asthmatic attacks.

Magnesium deficiency is widespread so increasing magnesium rich foods should be an essential part of the asthmatic's diet.

Good sources of magnesium are:

- Green leafy vegetables
- Nuts and seeds
- Beans – chickpeas and haricot, for example
- Legumes
- Dark chocolate

Magnesium can be absorbed through the skin and this characteristic is taken advantage of through Epsom salts baths.

The recommended daily allowance was 400mg daily but more recent recommendations say that the amount of magnesium that should be taken on a daily basis should be equivalent to the RDA for calcium. That is 800mg daily.

If you're unlikely to be able to take in enough foods containing magnesium, then supplementation should be considered. Magnesium is easy to source at most supermarkets and is economically priced.

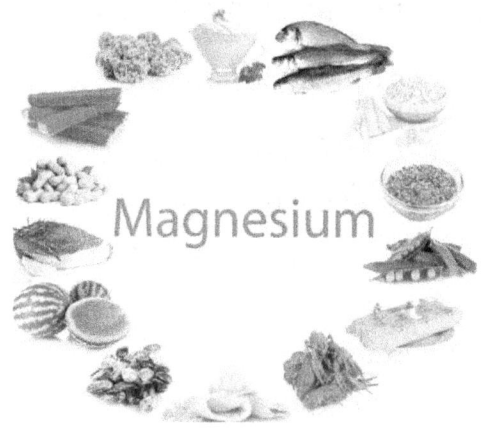

I have given a broad overview of magnesium but this seems a good place to look at it in more detail in relation to eosinophils. I have already mentioned eosinophils are cells found in the more severe and chronic forms of asthma. What is their function and what do they have to do with magnesium intake?

Eosinophils

I have already stated that the twitchiness found in the chronic, more severe, forms of asthma is mainly caused by eosinophils. To understand this a little more, it may be judicious to look at eosinophils in a little more detail.

Eosinophils are specialised immune system cells that are pro-inflammatory in nature. They contain granules in their cytoplasm that are filled with enzymes and protein.

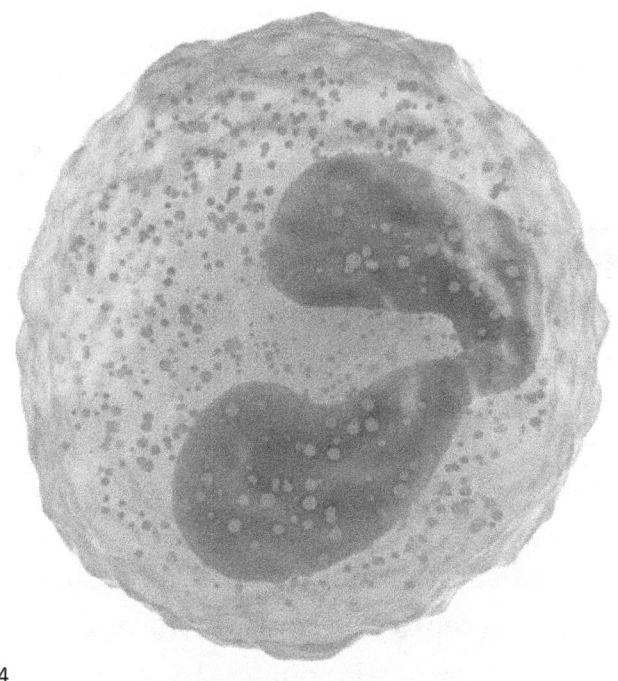

an eosinophil

They have many and diverse functions including:

- moving to inflamed areas
- trapping unwanted substances
- killing cells

---

[14] https://www.news-medical.net/life-sciences/Eosinophil-Function.aspx

- modulating the inflammatory response
- anti-bactericidal and anti-parasitic activity
- involvement in allergic response

This is all well and good but eosinophils, like many immune system cells, may be subject to inappropriate inactivation. They may accumulate and as such they contribute to the symptoms and disease process in allergic asthma.

The increase in eosinophilia may well be due, in part to a magnesium deficiency. Since it is now accepted that approximately 80% of the population are magnesium deficient it may be worth looking at this in a little more detail than we have already covered.

A magnesium deficiency – referred to as hypomagnesia – has been found, in experimental animals, to induce a number of immune system dysfunctions including:

- hyperaemia – an excess of blood in the vessels supplying an organ or other part

of the body leading to red, warm, painful and swollen areas.
- An increase in Immunoglobulin E which is involved in allergic actions
- Neutrophilia – an increase in neutrophils, circulating in the blood. Neutrophils are cells of the immune system
- **Eosinophilia – an abnormally high level of eosinophils circulating in the blood**
- An increase in cytokines which are pro-inflammatory in nature
- Mast cell degranulation – mast cells play an important part in wound healing, angiogenesis, defence against pathogens and protecting the blood brain barrier. However, they also induce some of the symptoms found in allergies.
- Histaminaemia - the presence of histamine circulating in the blood.
- Splenomegaly – abnormal enlargement of the spleen.

Given this information, it can be seen that many of the symptoms found in the chronic - and more severe types of asthma - may well be due to a magnesium deficiency and, following on from that, may be treated effectively by increasing foods, containing magnesium. In the diet.

Inflammation, free radicals and antioxidants

Free radicals are everywhere; we can't avoid them. They are generated from the metabolism of food that we eat and they are generated from:

- Cigarette smoke
- Cosmetics
- Air pollution
- Pesticides
- Radiation

Indeed, anything that involves chemicals including household cleaners and perfumes.

Free radicals, as we have already seen, are unpaired electrons. Electrons are stable when paired up but if they are unpaired or odd they form free radicals. They are formed when oxygen interacts with certain molecules. Like an out of control pinball free radicals dash around damaging anything that they come into contact with. When they crash into important cellular components such as cell membranes or DNA then serious damage or cell death can occur.

Free radical damage can be risk factors for asthma.

Antidotes to free radicals are antioxidants. Antioxidants are found in food but not the overcooked processed food that is often served up nowadays. When food is cooked most of the antioxidants are reduced or destroyed altogether. This does not mean that processed food does not have some benefit. It can still provide fibre, carbohydrates, fats, protein and some minerals. However, for the purposes of neutralising free radicals they do not offer much benefit for an inflammatory condition like asthma.

Antioxidants have to been taken in larger quantities than free radicals are being generated. This sounds difficult. We can make a guess that if the amount of processed food that we eat outweighs the non-processed food that we are not achieving our objective. However, we also have to take into consideration the external sources of free radicals such as household cleaners. We can now see that there is not much room for including processed food into the diet if we are trying to avoid damage to the cells and organs of our body.

Genetic propensity will play a role in which part of the body is most likely to be affected by free radicals.

There are a number of antioxidants that appear to have superior properties. These antioxidants are either minerals or vitamins.

The water soluble vitamins

The water soluble vitamins are the B and C vitamins. Vitamin C is probably one of the most well-known of the vitamins and most people know that it can be found in fresh fruit and vegetables. It is easily destroyed by heat whether this is by sunlight or cooking. As it is water soluble it easily leaches into the water that it is being cooked in. Any vitamin C that survives in the water is normally thrown away.

Vitamin C is a water soluble antioxidant and a powerful anti-inflammatory. Some studies have shown that asthmatics with low levels of vitamin C tend to have more flare ups of their condition.

Vitamin C is easily destroyed by heat and sunlight so fresh food should not be left for a long time. Cooking times should be as short as possible.

Vitamin C

Citrus fruits, green peppers, strawberries, tomatoes, broccoli and sweet and white potatoes are all excellent food sources of vitamin C (ascorbic acid)

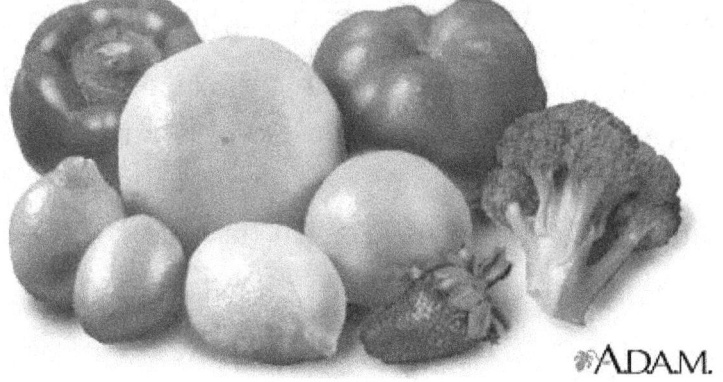

Vitamin C deserves further investigation because it is probably the best weapon that you have in relation to asthma. Firstly, though, you have to understand that the Recommended Daily Intake (RDI) of vitamin C which is 75mg for adult women and 90mg for men is woefully low. It was set at this amount as the minimum intake to prevent scurvy

The amount is nowhere near enough to prevent inflammation in the airways.

In 1974, the US Food and Nutrition board actually set the RDI at an unbelievable low of 45mg daily. While this amount may just prevent scurvy, it does not impact other areas that it is involved in, in any meaningful way; much higher amounts are needed for the immune system to be functioning at optimum speed.

It is well known that larger amounts of vitamin C can decrease the incidence and severity of the common cold. The form of vitamin C which I am writing about, is ascorbic acid and it is antiviral and antibacterial in nature.

It is required for the phagocytic activity of leukocytes which means that certain white immune system cells surround infective agents such as bacteria and ingest them.

This is a remarkable defence mechanism but only available if you are vitamin C sufficient.

Studies have also shown a 31% decrease in respiratory illness when 200mg of ascorbic acid is taken daily compared to a placebo. With a daily intake of 1000mg of ascorbic acid daily there was a 63% reduction of illness daily.

The recommendation is to take 3g daily for 3 days at the start of any illness.

A study showed that during a normal day on a normal diet there were 20ug per 10^8 of vitamin C but on day one of a cold it fell to 10^3 which was below the phagocytically effective level.

Adequate vitamin C prevents secondary bacterial infection due to common cold or stress.

Asthma exacerbations often during viral encephalitis, measles, mumps and chicken pox all of which respond very well – and in some cases prevent infection - to vitamin C.

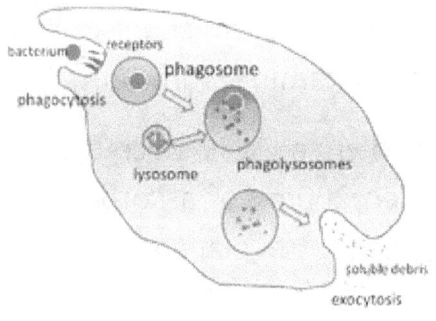

Note bacterium, being phagocytosed (red circle) into the heart of the cell where it will be totally destroyed. This action requires adequate amounts of vitamin C.

Full saturation of tissues is hardly ever achieved. In a book co-authored by Passmore of the British Panel on Recommended Allowances of Nutrition it stated:

The chief argument against the desirability of full saturation is that few people ever achieve it. It would need a revolution in British habits to eat sufficient fruit and vegetables to provide the vitamin at a level compatible to that needed by guinea pigs.

Indeed, the nutritionist Heisted stated that 'the term recommended allowance was adopted to avoid any implications of finality or……. Optimal requirements.

Vitamin C is also a very effective antioxidant pairing up with unpaired electrons so that they cannot damage tissues. It is certainly required when there is an inflammatory condition such as asthma as vitamin C is an effective anti-inflammatory.

A Thai study found that a vitamin C deficiency was a risk factor for asthma associated with severe asthma and decreased pulmonary function.

Here's the rub; most treatments including inhalers for asthma tend to diminish the vitamin C availability in the body.

Plant foods are rich sources of antioxidants. They can be found in all fruits and vegetables. Wholegrains are also a valuable source.

Specific antioxidants are:

- allium sulphur compounds – garlic, leeks and onions
- beta-carotene – mangoes, apricots, pumpkin, carrots, parsley, spinach and chard
- anthocyanins – berries, grapes and aubergine
- indoles – cruciferous vegetables
- copper – mainly sea food

- flavonoids- tea of all types, citrus fruits, onion, apple, red wine.
- Lignans – seeds and whole grains
- Isoflavonoids – soybeans, lentils, peas and milk
- Lycopene – water melon and tomato
- Selenium – lean meat and offal such as liver and kidney
- Nutritional yeast flakes are an excellent source of many antioxidants.

Other vital antioxidants

Zinc is a useful weapon in combatting inflammation caused by respiratory viruses. It has a powerful antiviral activity. Zinc supplementation alters airway inflammation and airway sensitivity. Zinc has further beneficial properties in that it stops many viruses from replicating.

A meta-analysis[15] of data from 17 studies found that children receiving zinc supplementation are

20% less likely to develop lower respiratory tract infections and pneumonia than those not taking zinc supplements.

The recommended dietary allowance of zinc is:

---

[15] Agarval R, et al Pediatrics 2007:119(6) 1120-30

Table 1: Recommended Dietary Allowances (RDAs) for Zinc [2]

Age	Male	Female	Pregnancy	Lactation
0–6 months	2 mg*	2 mg*		
7–12 months	3 mg	3 mg		
1–3 years	3 mg	3 mg		
4–8 years	5 mg	5 mg		
9–13 years	8 mg	8 mg		
14–18 years	11 mg	9 mg	12 mg	13 mg
19+ years	11 mg	8 mg	11 mg	12 mg

* Adequate Intake (AI)

Good sources of zinc are:

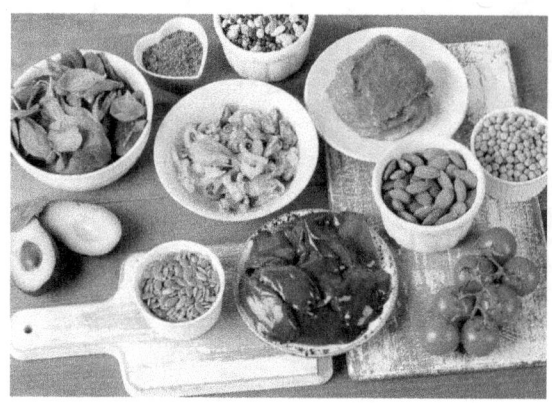

- Meat
- Shellfish
- Legumes – lentils, chickpeas and beans
- Seeds and nuts
- Dairy
- Eggs
- Whole grains

Sugar and inflammation

It has been known for a long time that sugar increases blood sugar levels rapidly and a number of negative effects occurs as a result.

1. When blood sugar rises there is a rise in pro-inflammatory molecules.
2. High blood sugar levels cause your body to produce molecules called advanced glycation end products. We normally shorten this to AGEs. These molecules also set off inflammation.
3. High blood sugar means that your cells become insulin resistant. This means that glucose is prevented from entering the cell. Apart from making people very tired, the sugar is then stored as visceral fat. This is the fat that is stored around the abdomen. Visceral fat produces lots of inflammatory molecules.

The main fuel of the brain is glucose but we need a supply of slow release carbohydrates that will provide fuel for cells without the rapid rise that causes insulin resistance.

Whole wheat foods are excellent in this respect. However, sugary sweets, cakes, biscuits, fruit juices, carbonated drinks are not. During the years of World War 2, sugar was in short supply. Cakes and puddings were mainly sweetened with grated carrot and coconut. A pint of rice pudding might contain one tablespoonful of sugar or sultanas to sweeten. This is far less than we find in desserts nowadays.

However, if the B vitamins are taken in high enough amounts – and they also tend to be deficient in diets – then the above negative impact of sugary foods tends not to occur.

The preferred source of energy for cells is glucose but it cannot be used unless there are sufficient B vitamins most notably thiamine, vitamin B1.

Thiamine is required to use glucose for cell energy. In fact, taking enough thiamine appears to reduce the need for diabetic medications. One such medication for diabetes, Metformin, has the unfortunate side effect of preventing thiamine's use in the body.

So can you have your cake and eat it? Well, yes, if you make sure that you have enough thiamine in your diet and magnesium. Magnesium is required to activate thiamine.

Like vitamin C, the Recommended Dietary Intake for thiamine is set at a woefully low amount of 1.4 mg.

Normally supplementation starts at 100mg (with 300mg of magnesium).

Fortified Nutritional yeast is an excellent source of B vitamins, including thiamine. Just two dessertspoons full of this sprinkled over food or into soups and stews after they have been taken off the heat goes a long way towards reaching optimum health.

The Omega three fatty acids EPA and DHA revisited

A recent study[16] reported that high dose supplementation of the omega3 polyunsaturated fatty acids, EPA and DHA in the third trimester of pregnancy significantly decrease the risk of persistent wheeze and asthma during the first 5 years of a child's life.

Other studies show that EPA and DHA significantly reduces asthma attacks if taken as a regular part of the diet.

The main sources of these two fatty acids are oily fish and walnuts.

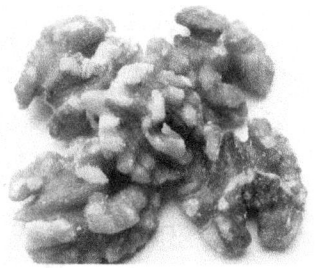

Walnuts are a great source of omega three fatty acids

However, studies do appear to show that it is the EPA fatty acid that exerts far greater effects on reducing inflammation out of the two. It targets the same pathway as steroid therapy

---

[16] https://www.ncbi.nlm.nih.gov/pmc/articles/PMC5831672/

but, of course, does not carry with it the same side effects.

Steroid therapy does carry great risks with its use. It raises blood sugar levels, thins skin, makes tendons and ligaments brittle, contributes to osteoporosis, lowers the immune system, damages muscles, causes psychosis and rapid weight gain among many other unwanted side effects. Some of these appear to be irreversible.

If this scenario can be avoided, then this it to everyone's advantage. I appreciate that not everyone likes eating fish or cod liver oil but there are many brands of orange flavoured cod liver oil that effectively disguise the taste we normally associate with this fish oil. There are many gelatine, capsuled supplements on the market, too. These are far more preferable to being prescribed steroids

Salicylates in food can contribute to asthma symptoms in some people.

Salicylates are chemicals found in plants which have pain- relieving, anti-pyretic and anti-inflammatory properties. They are naturally occurring in many fruit and vegetables and help to protect plants from being attacked by fungus. Salicylates are also found in aspirin.

There are a number of downsides to taking aspirin and salicylates. Some of the side effects of aspirin are the potential for indigestion, gastritis and ulcers. Salicylates may cause allergy type symptoms, in susceptible people. These include

- Asthma like symptoms – wheezing and trouble breathing
- Headaches
- Nasal congestion
- Changes in skin colour
- Itching, skin rash and hives
- Swelling of the hands, feet and face
- Stomach pain

However, if aspirin and salicylates are not a problem then they can be included as a treatment to reduce the inflammation found in asthma. Aspirin has excellent antioxidant activity but may damage the stomach lining in some susceptible people. Further, aspirin is well known for its ability to diminish vitamin C in the body.

Foods containing high amounts of salicylate are:

Fruit

Blackberry, blackcurrant, apricots, blueberry, dates, grapes, orange, pineapple, plum, strawberry, prunes, raspberry and sultana

Vegetables

Chilli peppers, courgette, green olives, peppers, radish and water chestnut

Seeds and nuts

Almonds, peanuts with skins on

Honey

Herbs, spices and condiments

Coconut oil, olive oil, basil, bay leaf, caraway, chilli powder, nutmeg, vanilla essence.

There is a very helpful website that produces a huge table of foods showing their salicylate value which can be found here:

https://www.sjhc.london.on.ca/sites/default/files/salicylate_free_diet_food_guide.pdf

Reducing salicylates will have an effect on asthma symptoms fairly rapidly if, indeed, that is a contributory cause.

As always detective work has to be employed. Even if there are three asthmatics in the family, the diversity of genes will mean that all can be affected for different reasons although there may be shared causes too.

The Asthma Imposter

Acetic acid has been found to cause allergic reactions in humans. Vinegar contains 5% of acetic acid so it is a dilute acetic acid and just adds flavour to food instead of causing the serious burns, it is capable of doing, when pure.

It is thought that acetic acid is capable of causing a syndrome known as 'reactive airways dysfunction' or RADS. This is due to its irritant effect.

This syndrome has similar characteristics to asthma. Symptoms include dyspnea, cough, wheezing. However, it differs in that exposure to tiny doses does not cause a reaction many weeks after its onset in the way that a true allergic reaction found in asthma would.

Another difference is that RADS is often characterised by prolonged wheezing and asthma type symptoms for a number of weeks after exposure. This would not occur –in true allergic asthma where exposure to an allergen would be of a much shorter duration. Not only is acetic acid implicated in RADS – and should be considered as a possible cause of asthma like symptoms but many other pollutants – gas and fumes, for example - can have the same effect and lead to long term disease of the airways.

It is important to understand that RADS is a non-immunologic reaction. There are also non-immunologic contact urticarias of the skin. Inflammatory reactions can appear within a short time after contact with the offending substance. These 'immediate-type irritancy' occurs without previous sensitisation.

Some individuals, who have not heard of RADS assume that the appearance of urticaria and asthma type symptoms must be due to an allergic response, when this is not the case.

People with RADS are unresponsive to asthma treatment. It is important, though, that the symptoms are treated quickly to avoid it becoming a chronic condition.

There was, for long enough, a lack of effective treatments and the outcome for many with RADS was poor.

However, studies[17] with high dose oral vitamin D supplementation of 2000 international units have proved highly effective.

Vitamin C at 1g-2g is also a good treatment for RADS.

Recognised Causal Agents[18]

Household – floor sealants, spray paint. Bleaching agents, household cleaners containing morpholene.

Chemical chlorine – sulphuric acid, ammonia, hydrochloric acid, acetic acid, phostene, hydrogen sulphide, sodium azide, sodium hypochlorite, toluene di-isocyanates, organic solvents

---

[17] https://www.ncbi.nlm.nih.gov/pmc/articles/PMC3196486/
[18] https://www.ncbi.nlm.nih.gov/pmc/articles/PMC3196486/#b1-jaa-4-087

Industry – paint spraying, metal-coat removers, welding, heated plastics or acids, epoxy resins, perfumes, pesticides, enzymes, industrial cleaning products, dust or mould in silos.

Other- fire and smoke inhalations, burning paint fumes, tear gas, locomotive exhaust, World Trade Center collapse in New York.

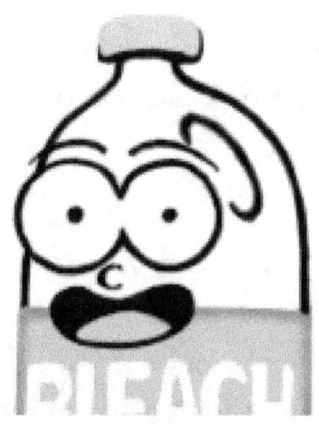

Inhaling fumes from household cleaners such as bleach can cause RADS.

Theophylline

Theophylline is a drug that is used to treat a number of respiratory disease such as asthma and chronic obstructive pulmonary disease (COPD). It has a number of therapeutic effects on respiratory health including:

- Relaxing bronchial smooth muscle and
- Having an anti-inflammatory effect

When muscles in the airways are relaxed then breathing becomes easier as they open up. Air can flow more easily. The tightness is alleviated.

Theophylline also reverses corticosteroid resistance. This is normally found in COPD and severe asthma. As such theophylline is often used as an adjunctive treatment alongside inhaled corticosteroids such as Fostair.

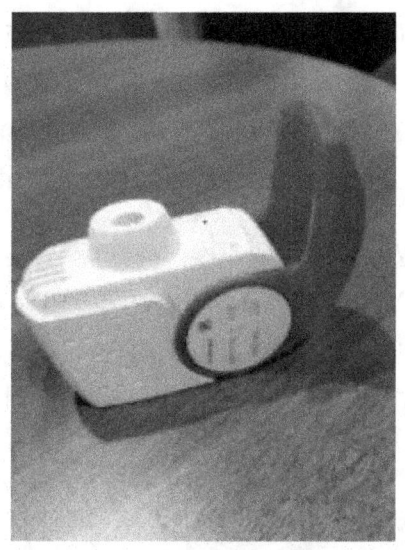

Fostair is a treatment for asthma

There are some patients for whom theophylline is contraindicated. These are those who have:

- Alcoholism
- Cystic fibrosis
- Those individuals who have medical conditions relating to the thyroid
- Diabetes
- Angina
- Have had a heart attack

The good news is that theophylline is found in cocoa in good amounts and therefore in dark chocolate- especially that which contains 85% solids. It is also found in lesser amounts in tea.

As theophylline is an adenosine antagonist then it has the potential to prevent sleep. Adenosine is a neurotransmitter that promotes sleep. It is found in Brewer's yeast, oily fish and lean meat.

Therefore, in order to address some of the issues found in respiratory disorders a mug of cocoa will be helpful but, instead of drinking it late night, it should be drunk in the morning where it will quickly help to open airways. Drinking chocolate is not suitable as it consists mainly of sugar and that is inflammatory. Dark chocolate with cocoa solids of 80% or more can be eaten and is generally one of the more enjoyable adjunctive treatments to respiratory diseases. Milk chocolate does not contain anywhere near therapeutic levels of theophylline and should not be eaten in preference to the high cocoa solid dark chocolate – as a treatment for respiratory disorders anyway.

Theophylline can build up in the presence of a viral infection. As such, it is not recommended that extra amounts of theophylline – other than those normally found in the diet – are taken.

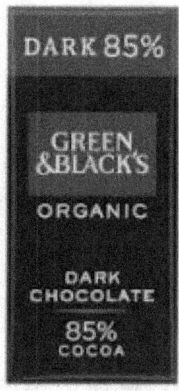

Dark chocolate with a high proportion of cocoa solids has useful amounts of theophylline.

As dark chocolate contains good amounts of magnesium then pairing it with high dose vitamin C will also enhance the impact of theophylline.

A strategic response to the state of acidosis in order to reduce pain and inflammation

Acidosis is implicated in many disease states yet very few people have heard of it or how it may impact health. However, the systemic acid-base balance may be responsible for significant changes in the immune response. Imbalances may help promote and prolong immune dysfunction. Acidic states may support certain infections increasing their severity and length.

There are different forms of acidosis – metabolic and respiratory - which may impact the immune system differently.

Metabolic acidosis can be further subdivided into types:

- lactic
- hyperchloraemic

Metabolic acidosis develops when too much acid is produced in the body or if the kidneys and lungs are unable to remove enough acid from the body. The pH of the blood should be around 7.4 and anything lower is referred to as acidosis whilst anything higher is referred to as alkalosis.

Lactic acid build-up – which is one of the subgroups of metabolic acidosis – occurs after prolonged exercise. It is responsible for the 'stitch' pain that we feel after intense exercise.

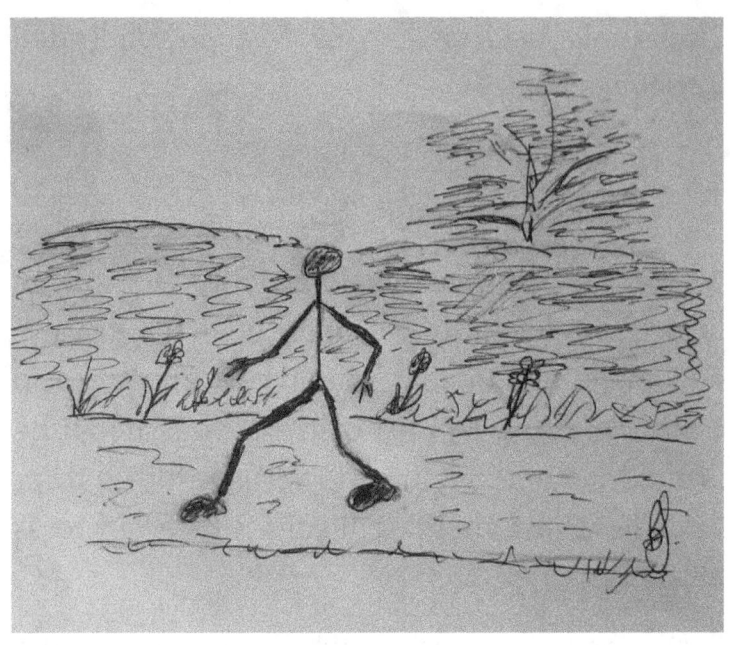

Intense or prolonged walking may result in lactic acid build up and metabolic acidosis

Hyperchloraemic acidosis occurs if when there is a decrease in bicarbonate concentration and an increase in chloride so that there is an imbalance of these two substances.

The bicarbonate can be lost for two main reasons:

- It may be lost from the gastrointestinal tract. One possible reason is that this may be due to the use of laxatives.
- a defect in the body which causes poor regeneration. For example, in chronic kidney disease the kidney loses its ability to synthesise ammonia, regenerate bicarbonate and excrete hydrogen ions.

Dietary causes of metabolic acidosis occur when there is an excess of fat or protein in the diet which is not balanced by bases such as calcium, potassium and magnesium. The acidic residues of protein produce subclinical or low grade metabolic acidosis.

Such a state may cause:

- kidney stone formation
- reduced bone mineral density and increased bone resorption
- loss of muscle mass

- chronic diseases such as type 2 diabetes, hypertension and non-alcoholic fatty liver disease

High blood sugar levels indicate that there is some form of insulin resistance or that the production of insulin is not adequate to allow glucose to enter the cells to be used as energy.

When insulin is inadequate then fats are broken down and form ketones which can be used as energy. This action can also produce a state of acidosis known as ketoacidosis.

Sodium chloride (salt) is reported to be an independent and causal factor for inducing metabolic syndrome. Salt is added in huge amounts to just about every tinned and packaged food item unless it has 'reduced salt' on the label. This will often then be sold at a grossly inflated price.

On many an occasion when I have investigated items masquerading as low salt, they are anything but.

We do need salt in our diet. It is vital for our health but there can also be too much of a good thing; as such it may cause imbalances in other electrolytes.

High salt diets are implicated in the progression of multiple sclerosis, for example.

The recommended daily dietary intake for salt, in adults, is one teaspoon per day. This equates to 2.4g of sodium.

In children it is age dependent:

1-3 years = 2g of salt daily (equivalent to 0.8g sodium)

4-6 years = 3g of salt daily (equivalent to 1.2g sodium)

Respiratory acidosis occurs when the lungs cannot remove enough carbon dioxide.

Excess carbon dioxide will cause the pH of the blood and body fluids to drop making them too acidic in the process.

Respiratory acidosis is caused by:

- Underlying disease such as asthma, COPD, sleep apnoea or pneumonia
- Conditions which can decrease the respiratory rate or inflation of the lungs. For example, obesity may prevent full expansion of the lungs.

Respiratory acidosis may cause symptoms such as:

- Anxiety
- Blurred vision
- Headache
- Agitation and restlessness
- Twitching
- Confusion

But this is not a definitive list.

As just about every chronic and/or painful condition will be underpinned by inflammatory processes, what can be done about it?

Researchers at the Medical College of Georgia discovered a nerve centre in a cell layer in the spleen that is responsible for the immune response and any inflammatory processes that occur throughout the body.

It is quelled by the addition of just 2g of bicarbonate of soda in half a glass of water for two weeks.

Bicarbonate of soda addresses metabolic acidosis and helps prevent the underlying and damaging inflammatory processes that accompany chronic conditions such as:

- Asthma
- Diabetes
- Obesity
- Arthritis

A report from the Netherlands in relation to asthma found that sodium bicarbonate (baking soda) reduced respiratory distress when given intravenously during a life threatening asthma flare up.

High blood acidity has a number unwanted effects in those with breathing disorders. It can:

- Reduce the effectiveness of beta agonist inhalers which are used to dilate the bronchioles.
- Cause the heart to contract more weakly
- cause rapid shallow breathing

The administration of sodium bicarbonate has been found to relieve bronchial spasm and allows the efficacy of bronchodilators once again.

Although there had been fears that the addition of sodium bicarbonate would raise blood carbon dioxide levels, this does not appear to be the case.

An analysis by Buysse and his team of 73 children with life threatening asthma found that the intravenous administration of sodium bicarbonate for those with acidosis resulted in a 'significant decrease in acidity' and further 16 patients experienced 'prompt improvements in respiratory disease and level of consciousness.

The anticipated increase of blood levels of carbon dioxide actually decreased significantly.

The researchers note that sodium bicarbonate was given to 14 patients in a last-ditch attempt to avoid putting them on a respirator, and only one of these subsequently required ventilation. All the patients survived.

Given these results, Buysse and her associates concluded that sodium bicarbonate was useful as an adjunctive treatment for life-threatening asthma.

Alongside asthma there are many comorbid conditions and these include:

- Rhinitis
- Sinusitis
- Gastro-oesophageal Reflux Disorder
- Obstructive sleep apnea
- Hormonal disorders
- diabetes

which can all be helped by the administration of sodium bicarbonate.

Following on from the connection between asthma and diabetes, individuals with type 2 diabetes have similar risk factors to those found in:

- obesity
- endothelial dysfunction
- vascular inflammation
- dyslipidaemia
- cardiovascular complications
- end stage renal disease
- hypertension
- depression
- thyroid gland disease
- chronic obstructive pulmonary disorder

Sodium bicarbonate is cheap and easily obtainable from any supermarket and can be found in the baking department.

It is a superb medicine and deserves a place in every household.

Acidosis from any origin reduces leptin which plays a role in regulating body weight. Some asthmatics may find exercise and therefore weight control, difficult.

When bicarbonate (HCO_3^-) levels are low the kidneys upregulate an enzyme known as glutaminase.

This triggers cortisol production and raises blood pressure. It follows that a high protein, high fat diet or a diet that raises the blood sugar levels beyond its capacity to cope through insulin's regulating function, will inevitably raise blood pressure.

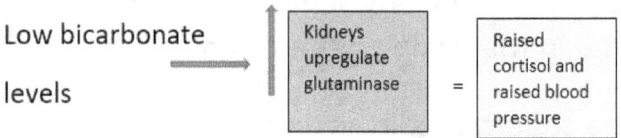

For those who like chemistry, it mediates this through the pituitary-adrenal cortex-renal glutaminase axis.

It has also been reported that upregulated cortisol bioactivity may be diet driven and promote insulin resistance in its wake.

Inflammation is implicated in asthma. It causes the lining of the airways to swell. It also helps produce mucus. Steroid inhalers may help with inflammation but as they increase blood sugar levels, they may also predispose to a pre-diabetic or diabetic state.

Extracellular acidosis helps the synthesis and release of inflammatory mediators especially tumour necrosis factor (TNF) and nitrous oxide (NO).

An alkaline diet – or the addition of sodium bicarbonate – decreases inflammation and increases growth hormone production. Thus it has anti-ageing effects.

The importance of optimum tissue pH can also be understood when you consider that the failure of local anaesthesia in inflamed tissue occurs when the tissue is in an acidic state.

Given that sodium bicarbonate can affect the severity, length and outcome of a disease, its worth should be more widely known. Indeed, in hospitals, it is often used intravenously to treat patients with severe conditions which have often worsened because they are in a state of metabolic acidosis which exacerbates the condition.

Pondering on this, this morning, I stated to my husband that we would be far better filling the salt pot up with sodium bicarbonate and sprinkling that on our meal.

Finally, and in relation to asthma and respiratory conditions, most respiratory bacteria and viruses thrive in acidic conditions. Thus by raising the pH of tissues, we can either prevent or reduce the impact of respiratory infection.

For long standing inflammatory conditions try:

Half a teaspoon of sodium bicarbonate in water twice a day for adults.

Continue for two weeks.

If the condition still hasn't cleared, reduce the daily intake to half of one teaspoon in water and sip throughout the day.

Continue this for one further week.

The inclusion of magnesium at 500mg daily would be helpful.

Children from 5 years upwards should have half the adult dose.

For immediate conditions. For example, you feel a virus or bacterial infection coming on, Arm and Hammer recommend:

6 X ½ teaspoonful taken in water at regular intervals throughout the first day.

4 X ½ teaspoonful taken in water at regular intervals throughout the second day

2 X ½ teaspoonful taken in water at regular intervals throughout the third day.

The Dangers of Manufactured Citric Acid (MCA)

As always, there can be more than one cause of any manifestation of a condition. During my research I happened to have my attention drawn to Manufactured Citric Acid and spent weeks following this through as it seemed to have implications for many chronic diseases such asthma, lymphoedema, lipoedema, Alzheimer's disease, arthritis, allergies and gastrointestinal disturbance. This is not a definitive list and it would not be unusual to find that an individual has a number of the above which appear, at first glance, to be unrelated.

Indeed, my attention was first turned towards the problems with MCA when I was advising someone on the benefits of real – not manufactured citric acid – in aiding gut motility.

The discovery of citric acid was credited to an alchemist Jabir ibn Hayaan going as far back at the 8th century. However, it was not isolated in its pure form until nine centuries later when Carl Steele crystallised it from lemon juice in 1784.

The lemon juice was imported from Italy and peak production occurred in 1915-1916 after which it began to decline due to cost.

The change from the crystallisation of citric to a fermentation process occurred in 1919 in Belgium using the mould known as penicillium. However, the duration of fermentation and the risk of contamination meant that the use of penicillium was abandoned.

In 1917, James Currie – an American food chemist – discovered that the mould *Aspergillus niger* could produce cost effective amounts of citric acid using molasses as the raw material.

In 1919, Pfizer adopted this method and began to produce citric acid using *Aspergillus niger*. This method is used today and we refer to this citric acid as manufactured citric acid or MCA.

The Food Standards Agency normally evaluates food additives for safety and they are given GRAS status – Generally Recognised as Safe. However, the Food Additives Amendment 1958 excluded any additives – including MCA – that were in use before 1958 that had not appeared to have demonstrated harm.

This does not mean that it does not cause harm. Some conditions take many years to diagnose and even so, the underlying cause may still be unknown.

99% of citric acid used today is the MCA sort. It is a ubiquitous substance and arguably the most common food additive. It is used to stabilise and preserve the active ingredients.

The global market growth and the related use of citric acid is undoubtedly driven by concomitant growth in pharmaceuticals, cosmetics and processed foods.

It can be found in:

Processed and prepared foods

Carbonated beverages, fruit and energy drinks

Nutritional supplements and vitamins

Common snacks

Confectionary

Pharmaceuticals

Canned fruit and veg

It is also used in non-food stuffs as it is a useful disinfectant against many viruses and bacteria.

Currently, the market share of MCA appears to be taken by:

Food and beverages	70%
Pharmaceuticals and cosmetics	20%
Cleaning and softening agents	10%

In a research paper[19] the potential harms of MCA are raised. The authors cite four case

---

[19] https://www.ncbi.nlm.nih.gov/pmc/articles/PMC6097542/

reports of individuals who demonstrate symptoms which include:

Joint pain with swelling and stiffness, muscular pain, dyspnea, abdominal cramping, and enervation that started within 2-12 hours of ingesting anything which contained MCA.

The severity of symptoms appears to be the deciding factor in how long before they resolve which could be anywhere from 8-72 hours.

The case participants did not know beforehand which foods contained MCA yet were able to correctly identify, based on symptoms, those which were.

It was found that the ingestion of natural forms of citric acid did not result in such symptoms.

Aspergillus niger is thermos tolerant and cannot be killed. Even when it is the end products is still pro-inflammatory. It is extremely likely that there are contaminants from production.

China is the largest producer of MCA and continues to expand as demand expects. Auto immune disorders and allergies have been found to be increasing in parallel.

Indeed, some of other conditions that appear to be related to MCA ingestion are:

ASD, juvenile idiopathic arthritis, fibromyalgia as well as allergies and angioedema type conditions and neurological conditions.

Late onset Alzheimer's disease is associated with reduced nicotinamide adenosine triphosphate (NAD) metabolism and an altered citric acid cycle also known as the TCA or the tricarboxylic acid cycle.

As it is MCA that is found in pharmaceutical drugs, then the impact of taking such drugs cannot be ignored.

Serious side effects are outlined[20] and include the citric acid which forms part of potassium citrate and sodium citrate too. This include numbness, tingly feeling, swelling or rapid weight gain, muscle twitching, cramps, fast or slow heartbeat, confusion, mood changes,

---

[20] https://www.uofmhealth.org/health-library/d03951a1

bloody or tarry stools, severe stomach pain, ongoing diarrhoea or seizures.

The cure for these diseases cannot be clearer – manufactured citric acid must be cut out of the diet. This is far easier said than done since when I looked at many of the convenience foods I have in for when I am too busy to cook, I find that most of them contain citric acid.

It does not say that it is MCA but it is the manufactured sort that is added. I even find that my ketchup contains it so unless I can find alternatives, I am relegated to making my own. I would enjoy this but I do not always have the time to do so. Batch cooking is possible but I do not always have the space to store everything that I need to batch cook to cover everything that I normally buy that I now find has MCA in.

I do know that if buy products that are 'free from' that they are likely to cost more. However, if I set this against the amount I might pay to buy pharmaceuticals to treat any symptoms arising from MCA then they are likely to be very cost effective indeed.

It is always worth removing MCA from the diet entirely for one week to ascertain the impact this has on your condition. The effects of MCA do not continue after 72 hours (unless you are constantly ingesting it) and so you have a relatively short time to wait to see if removing this substance would be beneficial.

As a little bit of research, it would be useful to log everything you eat over a short period to see how many food, drugs and drinks you are ingesting which contain MCA. Do not forget to include sodium and potassium citrate.

Wrapping it all up

We have learned about arachidonic acid and how it is used to synthesise leukotrienes that are implicated in the asthmatic condition. We have also learned that our diets have changed dramatically since the turn of the last century.

With the advent of allegedly 'healthy' oils we have lost one of our main sources of vitamin D in the form of saturated fat. In addition, we have introduced a pro-inflammatory substance in the form of these oils that, due to their ubiquitous state in most processed food, is eaten on a daily basis.

Our sugar consumption has increased far beyond what could reasonably be called acceptable. Sugar raises inflammatory levels.

Minerals that help reduce the severity of asthma attacks are, research shows, deficient in the majority of the population.

Our consumption of fish has reduced since the 1950's when it was not unknown for housewives to make fish head soup for a few pence.

As our diets change, a deficiency of some vitamins and minerals will occur while others may be found in excess. A deficiency of some may unleash a genetic potential which had been kept under reins by nutritional factors. If the diet is skewed to include different minerals, vitamins, fats and amino acids then it can change the course of a disease.

It is no surprise that many of the 'new' disease states rife in society at the moment began with the introduction of vegetable oils and the falling out of favour of nutrient rich saturated fats. Moreover, the addition of additives which have not been investigated for safety and derive from moulds are a major cause of concern especially when they are ubiquitous.

It is not surprising that many, once mild diseases, have now increased in quantity and severity.

We need to learn from this and return to healthier ways of eating. If we do not then the rates of asthma and other inflammatory conditions will continue to rise, not only burdening our health care systems but impacting on the quality of life and all that can be achieved if such conditions are not reined in through bespoke diet.

For every condition there **is** a bespoke diet.

Nutritional Formula for Respiratory Infection

Stopping infection using nutritional substances. This formula has been found to work in every case of respiratory infection regardless of the infective agent, stopping all symptoms within 48 hours maximum provided it is taken on day one of the symptoms of infection.

Children can have half the dose found below.

Day one – Must be taken at the first sign of infection	20,000 vitamin D + 1000mg of quercetin + 75-100mg of zinc	Vitamin D must always be taken with a little fat or oil in order to be absorbed properly
Day two and day three	5000-8000 IU's of vitamin D + 1000mg of quercetin and 75 - 100mg of zinc	The infection should be resolving at this point. If it is you can reduce the zinc to 50mg
Day 4 onwards – maintenance dose.	At least 2000 IU's vitamin D daily in the winter and all year around for the elderly (over 55 years) + 500mg -1000mg of quercetin daily + 50mg of zinc taken once weekly	

Vitamin C may be taken alongside the above starting in divided doses of 4000-5000mg on the first two days of infection and 500mg thereafter.

Adults take 3000mg of vitamin C for the first three days of a respiratory infection (children

1000mg) and then drop to half this dose if symptoms are beginning to dissipate.

Oregano oil is also a useful antibiotic and can be found online, in capsule form.

Take 25-50mg in divided doses daily.

The role of zinc deficiency in asthma

Both zinc and copper are needed for the optimal activity of the immune system. When we look at zinc we find it is involved in the synthesis of over 800 enzymes and macromolecules. A zinc deficiency is associated with both acute and chronic inflammatory respiratory conditions. While we expect some acute inflammation in order to deal with any present infection, chronic infection serves no useful purpose other than to further damage tissues and prevent healing.

Research conflicts about whether zinc supplementation is able to address asthma in children. This should not surprise us nor make us thrown the baby out with the bathwater.

There is generally more than one cause for an inflammatory reaction in the airways. Indeed, out of a hypothetical eight causes only four may be necessary to result in inflammation in the airways in the first individual while an entirely different two reasons only may need to be present in another. Genetics does allow for wide variation. Therefore, while zinc deficiency may contribute to asthma in some children, it clearly may not apply in others but we do not throw out valuable research because not every child reacts in exactly the same way.

Further studies[21] have found that zinc supplementation at 50mg/day did have a significant impact on lung functions as well as clinical symptoms. Other studies[22] have demonstrated a positive effect on asthma when vitamin C with zinc and omega 3 fatty acids were given to children. The combined therapy

---

[21] https://www.emro.who.int/emhj-vol-20-2014/volume-20-6/effect-of-zinc-supplementation-in-children-with-asthma-a-randomized-placebo-controlled-trial-in-northern-islamic-republic-of-iran.html#:~:text=It%20has%20been%20suggested%20that%20zinc%20deficiency%20can%20reduce%20antioxidant,of%20asthma%20attacks%20(23).

[22] Biltagi MA, Baset AA, Bassiouny M, Kasrawi MA, Attia M. Omega-3 fatty acids, vitamin C and Zn supplementation in asthmatic children: a randomized self-controlled study. Acta Paediatr. 2009 Apr;98(4):737-42. PMID:19154523 [Article retracted in Acta Paediatr. 2012 Aug;101(8):891].

was found to be more effective than a single therapy.

The children in the first study mentioned were found to have low serum levels of zinc and it is well recognised that allergic conditions are associated with a deficiency of trace elements which includes zinc as well as other like selenium. Wheeziness is also associated with a zinc deficiency.

The reasons given for the association between zinc deficiency and asthma are many. Some of these are that zinc deficiency:

Reduces the antioxidant capacity

Zinc is required to prevent virus from entering the host cell and a deficiency would impair this function so that infection – and accompanying – inflammation, could occur.

Other studies[23] also found that zinc supplements reduced inflammatory and airway hyper-responsiveness.

---

[23] Morgan CI, Ledford JR, Zhou P, Page K. Zinc supplementation alters airway inflammation and airway

Yet more studies[24] have suggested that zinc my increase the activity of the enzyme which is similar to that found in inhaled steroid therapy.

In these studies, IgE was not found to be a contributory factor. IgE is an immunoglobulin or antibody which is found in allergic reactions so one way of telling whether someone has an allergic or non-allergic asthma - the latter being classed as bronchial asthma- is to look at serum levels of immunoglobulins. There are 4 main types of immunoglobulins. These are: to describe their characteristics fairly simply are:

IgA – found in mucus membranes

IgE- found in allergic type responses

---

hyperresponsive-ness to a common allergen. J Inflamm (Lond). 2011; 8:36. PMID:22151973

[24] De Raeve HR, Thunnissen FB, Kaneko FT, Guo FH, Lewis M, Kavuru MS, et al. Decreased Cu, Zn-SOD activity in asthmatic airway epithelium: correction by inhaled corticosteroid in vivo. Am J Physiol. 1997 Jan;272(1 Pt 1): L148-54. PMID:9038914

IgG – found in infection

IgM – found in new non-specific infection

That is the simple version. Suffice to say that the above study did not find that serum levels of IgE decreased in the case group when zinc treatment had ended. This suggests that bronchial asthma is not driven by allergic responses.

Nevertheless, zinc does appear to inhibit the NF-kB pathway and so indirectly this does cause a decrease in serum IgE levels.

What is the strange sounding NF-kB pathway? This pathway is a protein transcription factor which helps to regulate your innate immunity (i.e. your 'general defence' immunity.) The NF-kB pathway links up signals from cells which imply pathogenicity in order to organise cellular resistance.

The conclusion of the above is that zinc is extremely helpful in those who have asthma and who additionally have asthma whether is it allergic in origin or not. However, those with bronchial asthma may be helped more The dosage used with zinc supplementation was 50mg/daily in children and lung function and clinical symptoms improved significantly.

When looking at zinc deficiency we have to consider which foods contain valuable amounts of zinc. Indeed, there are many but the latest diet fads which includes eating mainly plant based diets is not helpful. Phytic acid is found in plants and unfortunately it binds to zinc so that it cannot be absorbed in our digestive system.

All this nutrition that we take in and our bodies cannot use it. Phytic acid is known as an anti-nutrient and it is a good description. There are many anti-nutrients in plants some of which may be destroyed in cooking but then so will many of the vitamins that we require to keep us healthy including vitamin C and the B vitamins. Anti-nutrients are made in plants to prevent them from being eaten.

Here is a list of sources of zinc in mg/100g

Oysters – 70

Liver - 7.8

Dried brewer's yeast 7.8

Shellfish – 5.3

Meat in general – 4.3

Hard cheese 4.0

Eggs 1.5

Milk 1mg per cup

Factors reducing dietary zinc are:

Food refining and processing

Phytic acid

High dietary fibre intakes

Textured vegetable protein

Diuretics

Laxatives

Antacids

Deficiency symptoms which may accompany zinc deficiency asthma are:

Hair loss

Mental apathy

Eczema of face and hands

Infertility and defects in reproductive organs

Decreased growth rate

Post-natal depression

Congenital abnormalities

Loss of taste and smell

Susceptibility to infection in general

Zincs other functions are:

Growth

Insulin activity

Development of bones and skeleton in general

Development of the nervous system in general

Maintaining healthy liver function

Increasing appetite to healthy levels.

Medications which diminish vitamin C in the body

Inhalants, salicylates and systemic corticosteroids. (to a certain extent topical corticosteroids, too).

Aspirin

Beclomethasone

Budesonide

Hydrocortisone

Mometasone Fumarate

Trimcinolone

Dexamethasome

Flucatisone

Methylprednisolone

Prednisone

Diuretics (used in heart failure but lack of vitamin C, B vitamins and other nutrients flushed out by diuretics contribute to heart failure and inflammatory conditions like asthma.

Furosemide

Bumetamide

Torasemide

Bendroflumethiazole

Indapamide

spironolactone

Extra information

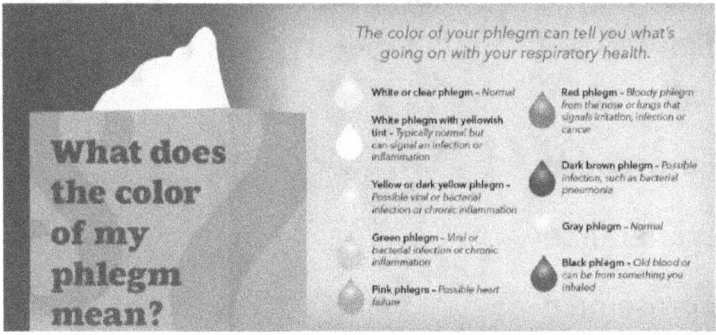

Protocol for bronchospasm, thick mucus

The dosage is for daily amounts:

200mcg of selenium (or 2 brazil nuts daily)

N-acetyl cysteine (NAC)[26] – a powerful antioxidant (please not there are various prescribing dosages. Children under two should not be given NAC but there is no harm in increasing foods containing L-Cysteine (see below for the list of common foods.

---

[25] https://www.unitypoint.org/news-and-articles/phlegm-cheat-sheet-recognizing-normal-and-concerning-colors-and-consistencies#:~:text=Phlegm%20from%20pneumonia%20can%20be,phlegm%20is%20from%20bacterial%20pneumonia.
[26] NAC is a metabolite – or end product – of cysteine.

Children and teenagers can be given 200mg NAC daily

Adults normally 600mg in divided doses but up to 900mg in divided doses has been suggested for severe cases.

Magnesium 300mg daily for adults.

65mg for children aged 1-3 years

110 mg for children aged 4-8

300 mg for those above 9 years

High dose vitamin C 2g-4g for adults/teenagers

Children 100mg and upwards until bowel tolerance is reached in 100mg hourly increments

Bowel tolerance may take a while to reach as vitamin C will be used up rapidly.

DMSO (low percent strength) rubbed over the affected parts including sinuses if needed)

Sit in hot steamy bath as humidity helps enormously or breathe in steam from a cup of coffee.

Coffee also helps expel mucus.

Foods containing L-cysteine

Eggs

Poultry

Beef

Whole grains

Yogurt and cottage cheese

Pork

Chickpeas, legumes, oats

Vegetables from the onion family

Mushrooms

Beef liver

Final message updated 06/09/2024

Huge amounts of vitamin c were the game changer for me. I no longer suffer infection, respiratory or otherwise and have not needed to use any inhaler or be prescribed steroids for years.

A percentage of the sales from these books goes to help charities like the one below.

The Exodus Project

My first introduction to the far reaching impact of The Exodus Project occurred when I was travelling around Cawthorne in one of their buses, visiting gardens. A young lad was happily munching on a sandwich. He looked up briefly, pointed to the driver and said,' He's my second dad, he is,' then he returned to his sandwich without further comment

Such remarks are often very telling and so I arranged to meet Jackie Peel and Martin Sawdon, at the charity's premises in

Barnsley. They set up the Exodus Project 20 years ago. They moved into their current premises – a redundant Methodist church - in 2010.

Both Jackie and Martin have been youth workers in their church. Martin worked in housing for the homeless in addition to working in learning disabilities services in institutional settings.

The work that the Exodus Project undertakes is of paramount importance to the communities it serves. These were former mining communities which became disadvantaged after pit-closures. Currently about 400 children attend mid-week activities from Monday to Thursday inclusive. These activities include dance, drama, craft, music, sports and games. In addition, there are weekend camps, cycle treks, outward bound activities, bowling and swimming. The children are taught valuable life skills including how to cook and bake. It is all about teaching children how to fulfil their potential and learn skills they will be able to pass onto the next generation.

The grounds, once overgrown, have been turned into a play- and camping - ground. A miniature railway is in the process of being installed.

Martin and Jackie have developed a unique model in that The Exodus Project goes beyond dispensing services. They are keen to build up relationships with the whole family and not just the child that attends the mid- week clubs. In addition, once children have reached the age of fourteen, they are invited to help out with the younger groups as junior volunteers. Once they reach the age of eighteen, they become adult volunteers. This model provides a constant supply of help from individuals who have benefitted already from attending such groups.

The building is large and inviting. It is decorated with bold colours and has comfy seating. It is a real home from home; a haven for families who have been disadvantaged by the closure of the life force of its community.

Martin and Jackie have clear ideas about how they wish to develop the Exodus Project but the lottery funding which they benefitted from is no longer available. Sadly, they have had to close two of their clubs due to lack of funding. This decision wasn't taken lightly. They do have two charity shops which raises some money and they obtain some funding from outside organisations for the use of their facilities. However, this is clearly not enough to keep their clubs, weekend activities and building going to cater for the ever growing number of children who are benefitting from the work being undertaken here. Neither does it allow for future development.

Exodus do have a Just Giving page which can be found here if you wish to help further their work https://www.justgiving.com/exodus

In addition, you can keep up with activities on their Facebook page here

https://www.facebook.com/search/top/?q=the%20exodus%20project%20barnsley&epa=SEARCH_BOX

If anyone wishes undertake an event like The Three Peaks - or run a marathon to raise funds for Exodus - then Martin or Jackie would be pleased to hear from you. This will enable their vital work in the community to continue. Contact them through their website to be found on www.exodusproject.org.uk.

For more books by this author look online at

https://www.amazon.co.uk/-/e/B07BPQZ5CD

https://www.amazon.com/-/e/B07BPQZ5CD

Some popular titles are:

Other books by this author include:

- **The EDS and Hypermobility Syndrome Diet**
- **Alleviating Symptoms of EDS**
- **Gastroparesis**
- **The EDS recipe book**
- **The Lipoedema Diet**
- **The Lymphoedema Diet: reverse and repair lymphatic damage**
- **The Anti-Virus Diet**
- **The Asthma Diet**
- **The Reluctant Bowel**
- **The MND Diet**

Among many others

They are available on Amazon

Lynne has written a semi-autobiographical trilogy.

While this trilogy is available on kindle and paperback on Amazon, it may be cheaper to buy from the link below.

They may be obtained off the publisher's website, in paperback form, where they are more reasonably priced.

https://www.shieldcrest.co.uk/?s=lynne+d+m+noble++

www.ingramcontent.com/pod-product-compliance
Lightning Source LLC
Chambersburg PA
CBHW060845220526
45466CB00003B/1243